MYTHS AND FACTS OF HIV/AIDS

Editor

Dr. KRITI GARG

Associate Professor,

Dept of Oral Medicine and Radiology

TANEESHA PUBLISHING

ISBN : 9788169244299
Edition : First, March 2026
Title : Myths and Facts of HIV/AIDS
Editor : Dr. Kriti Garg

Published by

TANEESHA PUBLISHING

An Imprint of **Taneesha and Prachi NextGen Publication**

Registered Address: Plot No. 48, Khasra No. 646, Road No. 2, Suman Nagar, Bahadarabad, Haridwar, Uttarakhand – 249402, India
Website : www.samantpublishing.com
E-mail : support@tpnextpub.com
Phone : +91 9760418103

Printed by :
Manipal Technologies Limited, Bengaluru - 560001, Karnataka

Co – Authors

Dr. Ibadat Jamil
Associate Professor, Dept of Prosthodontics

Dr. Shazia Aslam
Assistant Professor, Dept of Oral Medicine and Radiology

Dr. Sarika Umrao
Clinician at Dental Clinic

Dr. Ravi Seth
Associate Professor, Dept of Oral Pathology and Microbiology

Dr. Sunita Pathak,
Professor, Dept of Oral Pathology and Microbiology

Dr. Vishal Mehrotra
Professor & HOD, Dept of Oral Medicine and Radiology

Dr. Vinayak Rai
Assistant Professor, Dept of Oral Medicine and Radiology

TABLE OF CONTENTS

Chapter 1

INTRODUCTION

Dr. Ibadat Jamil

Acquired Immune Deficiency Syndrome (AIDS) is caused by the Human Immunodeficiency Virus (HIV). It is a critical disorder of the immune system which severely damages the body's normal defenses to infections. AIDS has emerged as a global crisis since its discovery in the summer of 1981 in the United States. Since the beginning of the epidemic more than 20years ago, over 60 million individuals have been infected by HIV worldwide and more than 20 million of them have died.

AIDS is the abbreviation for acquired immune deficiency syndrome. The disease is caused by virus known as human immunodeficiency virus.[11,80] The virus can remain in a person's body for many years without causing serious health problems.

DEFINITION: -

Acquired immune deficiency syndrome-AIDS was first defined by centre for disease control (CDC) Atlanta in 1982 as "a disease at least moderately predictive of a defect in cell mediated immunity, occurring in a person with no known cause, for diminished resistance to that disease."

1987 AIDS Definition: -

In August 1987, the CDC published a major revision of the adult case definition for surveillance, broadening the definition in three ways:

1. Inclusion of HIV encephalopathy and HIV wasting syndrome.

2. Inclusion of diagnoses made presumptively in cases with laboratory evidence for HIV infection.

3. Elimination of exclusions due to other causes of immunodeficiency in cases with laboratory evidence for HIV infection.

The main strategy for preventing the spread of AIDS-related diseases is still education in an effort to change high-risk behaviour. As new illnesses continue to spread throughout the world, success has been far from ideal. Communities and nations have been devastated as the fastest-growing HIV epidemic has moved from the homosexual to the heterosexual population; prostitution and the use of illicit recreational substances have been major contributing factors. There are numerous myths and theories about HIV and AIDS, but the best way to learn the truth is to seek information from trustworthy sources, including highly qualified professionals who specialise in HIV and AIDS management.

The only method to dispel any false information (or misconceptions) you may have heard is to become knowledgeable about HIV and AIDS. These facts on HIV and AIDS come from a number of trustworthy sources that are supported by scientific research. Doctors, nurses, counsellors, and other medical experts with expertise in HIV and AIDS are the most accessible sources of these.

What is a myth?

A myth is untrue or false information about something. Eventually, if these untruths are not shown to be false or untruthful, everyone starts to believe them. This can be dangerous, as people start believing the wrong information and the truth is ignored.

What is a fact?

A fact is the real, true information about something. A fact will dispell the myth or untrue information.

Some things you may have heard about HIV and AIDS but you're not sure whether they are true (fact) or false (myth)

Oral manifestations are the earliest and most important indicators of HIV infection. Oral health status of HIV positive individuals is in poor condition which may be a sequela of variety of factors. Oral lesions can not only indicate infection with HIV, they are also among the early clinical features of the infection and can predict progression of HIV disease to AIDS. Treatment of HIV patient involves trying to slow or stop the virus from spreading in the body's cells and treating or preventing disease that develop when a person's immune system has been damaged by the virus.

Chapter 2

HISTORY AND EPIDEMILOGY

Dr. Shazia Aslam

The CDC Morbidity and Mortality Weekly Report on June 5, 1981, contained the first description of AIDS. Five previously healthy, sexually active young gay males from Los Angeles were reported to have contracted Pneumocystis carinii pneumonia. This was swiftly followed by a case report of an uncommon and incredibly rare tumour called Kaposi's sarcoma in a gay male community in New York City.

The CDC received an increasing number of reports of comparable instances between June 1981 and May 1982. The illness was first known as "Gay-Related Immunodeficiency" since only homosexual and bisexual males were believed to be afflicted, and some feature of the gay lifestyle was assumed to be the likely source of the immunodeficiency. Subsequently, the CDC noted that heterosexual injecting drug users, Haitian immigrants, individuals with haemophilia, spouses, sexual partners, and children of individuals with the condition, as well as receivers of blood or blood components from infected individuals, have also been documented to have the same infection and tumour. The CDC named the illness AIDS in September 1982.While the number of cases was mounting in the United States, AIDS started appearing in Europe where an increasing phenomenon was observed. When investigators turned their attention to Africa they discovered an epidemic that could be traced through serologic studies to 1959.

HIV-1 was identified and named in stages. Not until early 1983 was there any indication that a human T-cell leukemia / lymphotropic virus might be the causative agent of AIDS. Luc Montagnier and scientists at the Institute Pasteur in France named the virus lymphadenopathy-associated virus. In the United States in May 1984, Robert Gallo and other investigators at the National Institute of Health reported the isolation of a group of cytopathic retroviruses and antibodies against those viruses in persons with AIDS. They termed it as human T-lymphtropic virus type III. At the same time, West Coast scientists at the University of California San Francisco who were studying the virus named it as AIDS associated retrovirus. In the summer of 1986, the international society on the taxonomy of viruses arbitrated changing the name to human immunodeficiency virus type-1. Montagnier and Gallo have been recognized as co discoverers of the virus.

EPIDEMIOLOGY

After being identified for the first time in the US, AIDS spread like wildfire within ten years. The majority of the world's regions have seen the diagnosis of AIDS cases, and the spread of HIV infection to some of the world's most populous places poses a threat to future AIDS case counts that are significantly higher than those that have been reported thus far. The lack of medical and public resources available in developed nations for diagnosis and reporting, political motivations that lead to a refusal to acknowledge the issue, and the challenge of estimating the extent of HIV spread when many infected individuals have not yet progressed to clinical disease have all hindered surveillance of the AIDS pandemic in many countries.

By June 30 1997 a cumulative total of 1,644,183 AIDS cases had been reported to the WHO. A report in December 1997 by the UNAIDS/WHO working group on Global HIV/AIDS and STD Surveillance revised the estimate of the number of adults and children living with HIV/AIDS upward to 30.6 million, nearly doubling their previous estimate.

The estimate of 30 million infected with HIV represents 1% worldwide of sexually active adults between the ages of 15 and 49 years. The projection for the number of persons living with HIV infection in the year 2000 was 40 million. The estimate of current incidence worldwide was 16,000 new infections per day during 1997. Most new infections were due to heterosexual transmission. It has been estimated that infant and child mortality in the major cities of the Americas, Western Europe and sub-Saharan cities Africa could be 30% greater than would have been expected without the AIDS epidemic.

The AIDS epidemic in Western Europe, Canada, New Zealand and Australia has shared many features of the epidemic in the United States. The estimate for new infections in Western Europe in 1997 is 30,000 and for the North America 44,000, totals less than the number of AIDS cases diagnosed in recent years.[97] Most cases from these geographic areas have been in homosexual/bisexual men with a significant minority among injection drug users, although Australia and New Zealand have had a relatively smaller epidemic in the drug-using population.

HIV/AIDS IN AFRICA

AIDS has taken its greatest toll in Sub-Saharan Africa. The WHO estimates that 16 million persons are living with HIV/AIDS in these areas, representing 2/3 of the world's total and 3% of the subcontinent's population. Most AIDS cases have been reported from central and eastern Africa.

HIV/AIDS IN ASIA

Between 1980 and 1990, only 855 cases were known in Asia. The first major epidemic occurred in Thailand and India followed by Vietnam, Myanmar and Cambodia. By the end of 1997, there were 69,000 AIDS cases in the region, representing an 80-fold increase from the last decade. Now 6.5 million are estimated to live with HIV/AIDS in Asia.

Chapter 3

ETIOLOGY & PATHOGENES

Dr. Sarika Umrao

The human immunodeficiency virus (HIV), a retrovirus, is believed to be the cause of AIDS. HIV-1 and HIV-2 are the two distinct forms of the virus. The principal causal viral agent, the human immunodeficiency virus type-1, was identified by researchers in 1984, three years after the first reports of a disease that would later be recognised as AIDS. A second strain of HIV, known as HIV-2, was discovered in a West African AIDS patient in 1986. AIDS and immunological degradation are caused by both viruses. HIV-1 and HIV-2 are linked to comparable opportunistic diseases and AIDS, and they share the same routes of transmission.

In persons infected with HIV-2, immunodeficiency seems to develop more slowly and to be milder. Compared with persons infected with HIV-1, those with HIV-2 are less infectious early in the course of the infection. As the disease advances, HIV-2 infectiousness seems to increase; however, compared with HIV-1 the duration of this infectiousness is shorter[19]: the median time from infection to AIDS has been reported to be approximately 10 years for those infected with HIV-1n but almost 20 years for those with HIV-2.

The AIDS virus is a retrovirus now called HIV-Human Immunodeficiency Virus. It belongs to lentivirus group called slow virus. Retroviral infections are characterized by the production of strong and prolonged humoral immune response in the host.

Based on their pathogenic potential, retroviruses are classified into three subfamilies:

1.Oncovirus, which includes human and animal retroviruses responsible for the induction of neoplastic diseases (HTLV-I, HTLV-II).

2. Lentivirinae, which are responsible for the induction of a variety of non-neoplastic disease in animals and humans (HIV-I, HIV-II).

3. Spumavirinae which have not yet been linked to any known disease.

In 1983, French researcher recovered reverse transcriptase, an enzyme responsible for transcribing RNA into DNA, in a lymph node from a man with signs and symptoms of what was known as lymphadenopathy syndrome, was recognized as an early manifestation of AIDS.

The identification of reverse transcriptase was the first indication that a virus, preserving its genetic information in the form of RNA, might be responsible for the immune deficiency described in affected individuals. The presence of reverse transcriptase, together with signs and symptoms of the disease also suggested that the causative agent of AIDS belonged to a family of viruses called retroviruses. After the initial recovery of viruses from lymph nodes, HIV was isolated from peripheral blood mononuclear cells both in patients with clinical manifestations of AIDS as well as in patients without any clinical signs or symptoms.

HIV PARTICLES: -

HIV-1 virions comprise a nucleoprotein core surrounded by a lipid bilayer containing the viral surface (gp120) and transmembrane (gp41) envelope proteins. Gp120 contains viral determinants that bind to host cell surface receptors. Gp41 contains an N-terminal hydrophobic domain, which is thought to initiate the process of virus cell membrane fusion, and also the transmembrane and cytoplasmic tail domains that anchor envelope in the viral lipid bilayer. The nucleoproteins core of the virions comprises two copies of viral genomic RNA and associated t-RNA molecules, along with mature gag and pol protein products. The matrix gag protein is believed to be associated with the inner leaflet of the lipid bilayer; the capsid gag protein forms the structural core of the viral nucleoprotein complexes and the nucleocapsid gag protein selectively binds viral genomic RNA. The mature pol proteins are virus associated enzymes PR, RT and IN.HIV-1 particles also contain the viral proteins Vpr and Vif. It has also been proposed that the viral Nef protein is incorporated by HIV-1particles. The host cell protein cycllophilin A is incorporated into HIV-1 particles by an interaction with the CA protein and is important for productive viral replication.

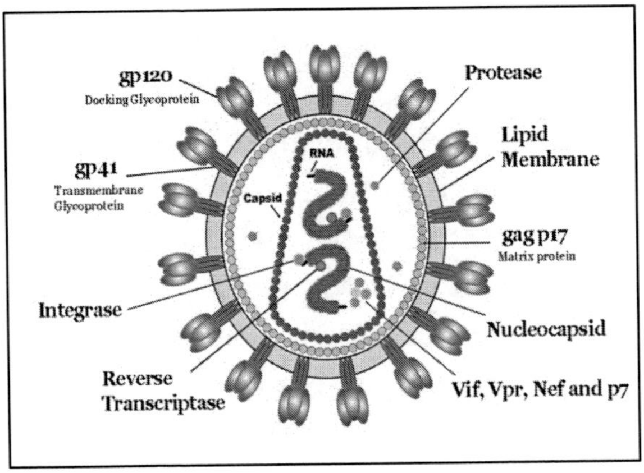

Figure -1: HIV particle

HIV GENES AND GENE EXPRESSION

The integrated form of HIV-1 also known as the provirus. Both ends of the provirus are flanked by a repeated sequence known as the long terminal repeats. The genes of HIV are located in the central region of the proviral DNA and encode at least nine proteins. These proteins are divided into three classes:

a) The major structural proteins: gag, pol and env

b) The regulatory proteins: tat and rev

c) The accessory proteins: Vpu, Vpr, Vif and Nef

PATHOGENESIS: -

HIV infection is essentially 100% fatal. The consequence of this viral lethality is based on the fact that HIV can directly attack cells of immune system, more specifically T-lymphocytes and macrophages. This initiates an essential irreversible immune suppression, leading to AIDS defining opportunistic infections and malignancies.

Two glycoprotein's gp41 and gp120 are subunits generated by the cleavage of the gp160 precursor. HIV target cells expressing CD4molecules, particularly CD4+ T lymphocytes, monocytes and macrophages taking advantage of the affinity between the viral gp 120 and the cellular CD receptor. The binding of gp 120 to CD4 receptors causes a conformational change in gp 120, which expose and stabilizes a cellular chemokine receptor called CCR5. These interactions activate gp41, resulting in fusion of the viral membrane with the cellular membrane which allows the viral RNA and reverse transcriptase transcribes the viral RNA into DNA, which integrates into target cell's genome. With the successful integration of viral DNA into the cellular genetic material, an infection has occurred. HIV gains entry into the body directly through the blood or at mucosal surfaces. The virus establishes itself within lymphoid tissues, where it replicates, makes itself available to the cells of the immune system and slowly brings about the destruction of the lymphoid tissue. Contact between the mucosal surfaces and HIV can result in infection of Langerhans' cells after only a couple of hours. Within a few days, the virus can be detected in regional lymph nodes. The rapid replication of HIV results in an initial viremia causing seeding of the virus to lymphoid tissue throughout the body. It is estimated that more than 10 billion virions with a half-life of approximately 1.6 days are produced daily in infected individuals.

Activated CD4+ lymphocytes express high levels of chemokine receptors and are primary targets of HIV. However, although these activated cells usually die within a few days. A latent reservoir of HIV is established among CD4+ cells. The initial control of viral replication is associated with antibody –dependent cellular cytotoxicity activity and HIV specific cytotoxic T lymphocytes. The hallmark of HIV disease is the progressive loss of CD4+ lymphocytes. Without intervention an average of 60 to 80 cells/mm^3 are lost every year; this loss is highly variable and occurs in periods of more stability and rapid decline. The lower the CD4 cell count the more susceptible is a patient to develop opportunistic infections.

Chapter 4

TRANSMISSSION OF HIV

Dr. Ravi Seth

The amount of HIV infection in a given bodily fluid, the virus's virulence, the fluid's capacity to permeate skin and mucosa, and the degree of contact with infected fluid are some of the factors that affect successful HIV transmission. Early in the epidemic, it was recognised that HIV could spread through intimate sexual contact and contaminated blood.

MODES OF HIV TRANSMISSION: -

1) DOCUMENTED MODES OF TRANSMISSION

A Sexual transmission

B Exposure to blood and blood products

C Vertical transmission from mother to fetus/child

D Injection Drug Users

E Health Care Workers

2) UNDOCUMENTED MODES OF TRANSMISSION

A Saliva

B Aerosol

C Dental rotary instruments

D Tears

E Urine

F Sweat

G Hepatitis B Vaccine

H Insect Bites

I Casual Contact

SEXUAL TRANSMISSION

AIDS was described as a sexually transmitted disease. In the early 1980s mainly homosexual/bisexual men were thought to be infected but over a decade later we know that majority of infections worldwide occur via intimate heterosexual contacts.

Due to trauma and subsequent abrasions of the rectal mucosa, as well as direct HIV infection of the bowel mucosa with infected semen (semen with 10 to 50 infectious particles per millilitre has a higher concentration of infectious viruses than vaginal fluid), anal receptive intercourse is linked to a high degree of risk for HIV transmission. The seminal fluid may include 0.01% to 5% of infectious cells.

Venereal disease not only increases the number of inflammatory cells infected with HIV, enhancing viral replication but cause breaks in mucosa facilitating entry of the virus into the body. Studies in the United States have supported this finding, where the presence of venereal disease such as herpes simplex virus and syphilis has been associated with an increased risk for HIV transmission among heterosexual couples.

Vaginal mucosal cells may be directly infected by HIV increasing the risk for infections in women. However, anal intercourse and bleeding as a result of intercourse are major determinants for heterosexual sexual transmission of HIV to women. However, genital tract secretion of HIV increases in infected women who use oral contraceptives rendering these women more able to transmit the virus during heterosexual intercourse.

Transmission of HIV during oral intercourse between men; although these reports are anecdotal unprotected oral-receptive intercourse cannot be considered safe until other risk factors facilitating transmission by this route.

BLOOD

Infected individuals carry HIV within infected cells and as a free virus. Free HIV has been isolated in quantities of 1 to 5000 infectious particles per milliliter of plasma. Individuals with more advanced stages of disease and during the first couple of weeks after infection will show a high concentration of infectious viruses. HIV is found in even greater numbers with in infected cells than as free viruses in the plasma.

HIV may be present in 1 in 10 to 1000 peripheral blood mononuclear cells in infected people. Moreover, thousands of infectious viruses can be produced and harboured by each infected cell. HIV serum concentrations are significantly lower in asymptomatic people than in symptomatic people and patients with more advanced stages of the illness.

The high concentration of HIV in plasma makes this fluid one of the principal routes of transmission of HIV. Regular laboratory tests to detect infectious agents, other safety measures such as viral inactivation factors are being used the estimated risk of contracting HIV disease from a blood transfusion is 0.0025% to 0.0003% per unit transfused.

BLOOD PRODUCTS

Blood products are used for patients with specific factor deficiencies such as factor VIII, factor IX and von Willebrand factor. Components of whole blood such as red blood cells, plasma cryoprecipitate or platelets, coagulation factors are extracted from plasma and cryoprecipitate from pools of thousands of donors increases the risk of undetectable HIV.

MOTHER TO NEWBORN

Vertical transmission has been the principal cause around 80-90% of HIV-1 infection in children.[138] It is estimated that infected mothers transmit the virus on an average of 30% to their newborns with numbers ranging from 7% to 71%. The highest risk, 71% was associated with the presence of maternal p24 antigenemia. The risk for perinatal transmission was estimated to be 50% in mothers with CD8+ cell counts of at least 1,800 cells/mm^3 and 29% in women with CD4+ cell counts below 600 cells/mm^3.

It is not clear how or when transmission of HIV from the mother to the child occurs. HIV has been found in placentas and fetuses and has been isolated from cord blood and amniotic fluid supporting inutero transmission. However, in some instances HIV cannot be isolated from cord blood but is recovered in infants who were infected but were older than one month.

Data showing that only one monozygotic twin may be infected but that the firstborn of twins has a higher risk of infection further supports the idea that HIV transmission during delivery is linked to contact between the mother's blood, genital secretions, or amniotic fluid and the newborn. Babies who were exclusively breastfed had a 45% decreased incidence of postnatal mother-to-child HIV transmission at three months of age compared to those who were fed a combination of breast milk and formula or breast milk and other foods or liquids. Additionally, a high salt content in breast milk was linked to high HIV-positive women's. Additionally, a high salt concentration in breast milk was linked to an increased vertical transmission rate and a high breast milk viral load in HIV-positive mothers.

INJECTION DRUG USERS

The main way that HIV is spread among injectable drug users is through injection paraphernalia that has been contaminated by HIV-positive blood and then reused by an uninfected injectable drug user. High-risk sexual behaviour, sharing injection equipment, and frequent drug injection are drug-related behaviours linked to an elevated risk of HIV infection in the US and Europe. Sharing syringes, needles, and other injectable supplies is the biggest risk factor. Globally, injectable drug users frequently share. Another risk element is sharing with several injection partners.

Studies consistently demonstrate that a significant risk factor for HIV infection is drug use at "Shooting Galleries" sites where drugs are sold and injection equipment is made available for rental or sharing. Needle sharing frequency, the number of partners with whom paraphernalia are shared, the probability that those partners are HIV infected and the manner in which sharing occurs influence HIV risk. Other specific drug sharing practices also increases the risk of acquiring HIV, Frontloading is a practice in which an IDU uses a syringe to measure out a quantity of drug for someone else's use and then squirts the drug directly into that person's apparatus.

Additionally, any parenteral exposure might result in injection equipment contamination and subsequent HIV transmission; neither needle sharing partner's intravenous puncture is necessary. HIV can also be spread by subcutaneous or intramuscular drug usage. Cocaine usage, whether injected or smoked as crack, is linked to increased HIV infection rates in the United States. After adjusting for length of drug use, intravenous cocaine usage, and STDs, frequent trading of sex for drugs or cash is an independent risk factor for HIV infection among female injectable drug users. Homo-sexual and bisexual male injection drug users are at particularly high risk for HIV infection not only via sexual transmission but also because of high-risk prevalence of HIV in their needle-sharing peer group.

HEALTH CARE WORKERS

Transmission of the HIV infection to health care workers in an occupational setting is fortunately not a common event.[97]The cumulative risk to a health care provider for occupational HIV infection depends on following probabilities:

(a) the exposure will involve HIV

(b) infection to the health care worker will result

Of these first is the most amenable to intervention and it varies with occupation, experience skill, technique and infection control procedures. Most occupational HIV infections were caused by accidental injuries inflicted by needles or other sharp objects.

SALIVA

Both free virus and virus infected cells can be found in saliva.

However less than 10% of samples yield HIV and in concentration less than one infected virus per milliliter.[74]Saliva in itself is not considered an infectious fluid except during dental procedures when blood may mix with saliva.[74] But using PCR technique HIV proviral DNA can be detected both in individuals glandular secretions and in whole saliva. Culture attempts have generally placed the isolation proportion at under 5% with the exception of a 21% positively for low levels of virus.

If saliva is considered an infectious fluid we could except that under circumstances of spontaneous bleeding in the oral cavity a higher concentration of HIV should be present in saliva. Although high levels of HIV existed in the plasma, infectious HIV could not be detected in the saliva, even in the presence of severe periodontal disease and visible blood. Saliva plays an insignificant, if any role in HIV transmission.

DENTAL HANDPIECES

Potential cross contamination of HIV with dental hand piece has been considered. Results from various studies shows that human materials as well as HIV DNA can contaminate the inside of both prophylaxis angles and high speed hand piece.

AEROSOL

Aerosolization of infectious human papilloma virus has been documented during removal of warts with the carbon di-oxide laser and with electro-coagulation. However preliminary data from a study conducted in a clinical dental sitting did not indicate survival of HIV-1 in aerosol generated by high speed hand pieces, cavtrons or Nd:Yag lasers.

TEARS

HIV has been isolated from tears as well as from contact worn by infected individuals. According to CDC 1985 due to the possibility of the extremely low concentration of HIV in tears, less than one infected virus per milliliter.

URINE

HIV has been recovered from the urine of infected individuals although fluid has never been implicated in the transmission of the virus.

SWEAT

Sweat has never been implicated in HIV transmission and probably does not contain infectious particles.

HEPATITIS B VACCINE

An initial hepatitis B vaccine was developed from plasma donated by a large cohort of homosexual/bisexual men but because of concerns of the recipients that HIV transmission may occur via this route, recombinant vaccines were developed. Concerns about an association between the initial vaccine and HIV transmission were not warranted since the process to develop this vaccine removes and inactivates HIV.

INSECT BITE

Theoretically transmission through biting or blood sucking insects could occur if the virus can multiply within the insects or survives in the mouthpiece of the insect, enabling a mechanical spread of the virus.

In African insects DNA sequences homologus to HIV have been found but there is no evidence indicating that free virus or viral replication can survive inside arthropode. Mechanical transmission of HIV was assessed in the experiments where mosquitoes and bedbugs gorged on HIV contaminated blood. Even with concentrations 100 times that found in individuals with HIV transmission from the insects could not be accomplished.

Chapter 5

MYTHS & FACTS OF HIV/AIDS

Dr. Kriti Garg

There are many myths about HIV and AIDS. Some of these lead to unfair actions by others and stigma.

Myth: My employer can force me to have an HIV test.

Fact: Only you have the right to decide whether to go for the test or not. Nobody, not even your healthcare professional, can force you to have the test, nor can anybody conduct the test without your permission.

Myth: My employer can fire me if I am HIV positive.

Fact: The outcome of your HIV test is confidential and only you and your healthcare professional will know the results. It's against the law for any healthcare professional to tell anyone the result without your permission. If you decide to tell your employer your result, he or she cannot fire you simply because you are HIV positive. Labour laws protect you. You should also ensure that you are familiar with your company's HIV policy.

Myth: It is safer not to go for an HIV test because you don't want people to find out.

Fact: It is important to have an HIV test to establish your HIV status. It gives you the power to take control of your life and make healthy lifestyle changes, whether you test positive or not. It's better to find out you are HIV positive at an early stage because, with the right care and treatment, you can live a long, healthy life. Always remember that your results are confidential, so people will only know if you tell them.

Myth: HIV-positive people don't live longer than three years.

Fact: HIV-positive people who take good care of themselves and receive good medical care can live for a long time with HIV. Healthy eating, good emotional support and the right medication can help the person live a long, healthy life.

Myth: You can tell that a person has HIV by looking at them

Fact: People who have HIV may not show any signs for many years. This is particularly true when the HIV-positive person looks after their health and follows healthy lifestyle choices.

Myth: HIV is a 'gay' disease and only gay (homosexual) people get HIV and AIDS.

Fact: HIV is spread through unprotected sex between gay (homosexual) people as well as people of the opposite sex (heterosexual). The main way the virus is spread in South Africa is through heterosexual sex. HIV does not discriminate against any person, regardless of their race or sexual orientation and socio-economic status.

Myth: You can contract HIV by touching an HIV-positive person

Fact: You cannot contract HIV by touching another person, unless you touch an open wound or are exposed to HIV- infected body fluids such as blood, semen and vaginal secretions and breast milk. HIV is passed from one person to another by:

- Having unprotected sex with an HIV-positive person
- Sharing infected needles and other sharp objects with an HIV-positive person
- Breastfeeding
- Direct contact with HIV-infected blood through open sores on the skin.

Myth: HIV medication (antiretrovirals) are a cure for HIV and AIDS.

Fact: There is no cure for HIV and AIDS. HIV medication only helps slow down the progress of the disease by stopping the virus from spreading in the body. Even though you cannot cure HIV, you can lead a healthy and longer life by managing the virus with the right treatment and looking after yourself both physically and emotionally.

Myth: There are traditional and herbal medications that can help treat HIV.

Fact: The only medications that have been proven to treat HIV and AIDS are antiretrovirals. These medications are registered with the Medicines Control Council, which is the organization that controls all medication in South Africa. While there is a place in South Africa for traditional medication, there is no evidence that these are effective in the treatment of HIV and AIDS.

Myth: Men are at a lower risk of getting HIV through unprotected sex than women

Fact: Even though there is now a link that HIV is reduced in men who are circumcised, anybody who has unprotected sex with an HIV-positive person is at risk of contracting HIV. HIV does not discriminate against people, regardless of their sex. The only way to reduce your risk of getting HIV is to always use a condom when having sex and by staying in a committed relationship with one partner only.

Myth: You can't contract HIV if you bath or shower after having unprotected sex with an HIV-positive person.

Fact: The only way a person can avoid contracting HIV is by not having sex at all or by using a condom when having sex with an HIV-positive person. HIV is passed into the body through body fluids such as blood, semen and vaginal secretions and breast milk. HIV cannot be washed away once the virus has entered the body.

Myth: People with HIV cannot work.

Fact: HIV-positive people can carry on working and contribute in a meaningful way to their families and broader society, as long as they look after their health.

Myth: HIV-positive people cannot have sex with their partner.

Fact: HIV-positive people can continue to be intimate with their partners. However, to protect against the spread of HIV, they must practice safe sex. This means always using a condom when having sex and staying faithful to one partner only.

Myth: It's better not to speak to children about HIV.

Fact: Adults sometimes believe it is better to protect children from the truth, but it shouldn't be so when it comes to HIV and AIDS. Providing children with all the information about HIV and how it's passed on, will help them to protect themselves against the virus, for example starting off by not touching blood on open wounds.

Myth: Red Ribbon is an AIDS symbol, sign of danger.[2]

Fact: Red Ribbon was conceived in 1991 by a group of artists in the United States of America who wants to draw attention to AIDS. Since then Red Ribbon has become an international symbol of AIDS awareness and visual expression of support for people affected by AIDS.

Myth: People who wear the Red Ribbon are infected with the AIDS virus.

Fact: People who wear Red Ribbon show their concern and support for people living with HIV &AIDS. By wearing the Red Ribbon, they are simply demonstrating their commitment to spread awareness and help fight the stigma and discrimination associated with HIV&AIDS.

Myth: You don't need HIV &AIDS awareness.

Fact: Young people are especially vulnerable to HIV infection because of a variety of factors such as curiosity, experimentation and most importantly peer pressure.

Myth: AIDS is mainly a problem of uneducated people especially living in the urban slums.

Fact: AIDS is everybody's problem. It cuts across community, caste, class, religion, education and occupation. HIV does not discriminate between educated and uneducated people.

Myth: HIV &AIDS are one and the same thing.

Fact: HIV stands for Human Immunodeficiency Virus. The virus can be transmitted from person to person; it decreases body's ability to fight against various infections leads to AIDS, which stands for Acquired Immune Deficiency Syndrome. HIV is the cause and AIDS is the effect.

Myth: It takes years for the symptoms of AIDS to develop, so there is no point in telling others about the infection.

Fact: It is true that it takes many years (8-10 years without treatment) after initial infection with HIV for the symptoms of AIDS to develop. It is very important to talk about it with your partner, and your partner should also be tested. It is the responsibility of a HIV positive person to avoid infecting others.

Myth: I can tell by looking at a person if she/he having HIV.

Fact: You cannot tell whether a person has HIV or not by looking at his/her appearance. There are no specific signs and symptoms of HIV infection for a long time. An infected person may look healthy and only a blood test for HIV can show whether a person is infected or not.

Myth: AIDS is a glamour business; so many celebrities are associated with it.

Fact: AIDS is not a glamour business. Some celebrities have associated themselves with the cause because of the seriousness of the disease.

Myth: Only female sex workers spread HIV infection.

Fact: Not only Sex workers, but anyone, male or female, can spread HIV. HIV mainly spreads through sex with an infected partner or multiple partners.

Myth: Sex with known person such as a friend or neighbor is safe.

Fact: Unprotected sex with anyone is not safe. No one can be guaranteed to be free of HIV, either neighbor or friend.

Myth: Only people with multiple sexual partners contract HIV.

Fact: People with multiple sexual partners are at a higher risk of getting HIV infection. Even a single act of unprotected sex with an infected partner may lead to HIV infection.

Myth: Oral sex is safe, because there is no penetration.

Fact: Oral sex is not completely safe. There is a low risk associated with it as compared to unprotected vaginal or oral sex. Unprotected oral sex can lead to HIV infection if either of the partners is infected with HIV and has sores or cuts in the mouth.

Myth: It is safe to have sex during menstruation, no chance of pregnancy and HIV.

Fact: It is possible, although not common, for a woman to become pregnant during menstruation. But there is definitely a possibility of getting transmitting HIV during menstruation.

Myth: It is safe for a HIV positive person to have unprotected sex with other HIV positive person.

Fact: HIV is of more than one type HIV-1 and HIV-2 and has different strains. It is possible to get infected with another type of stain during unprotected sex. Therefore, it is important for each of the HIV positive partners to avoid unprotected sex.

Myth: There is no risk of getting HIV with woman who charges a hefty amount for sex.

Fact: HIV does not differentiate between rich and poor; it is the behavior that puts you at risk.

Myth: Blood donation can lead to HIV infection.

Fact: Blood donation cannot lead to HIV infection, because the blood collection equipment is sterilized and not reusable.

Myth: The "Window Period" is the time when one has not tested positive for HIV, so it cannot be transmitted to anyone else.

Fact: When the body is infected with HIV, it takes 3-12 weeks from the date of exposure to HIV antibodies to appear in the blood. If the HIV antibody test is taken during the Window Period, it will give negative result, but the person may already the HIV infected and capable of transmitting the infection to others.

Myth: Cleaning a needle with hot water makes it safe for reuse and share.

Fact: Just cleaning a needle with hot water cannot prevent HIV; needle should have to be boiled for at least 20 minutes to sterilize them completely before using. Sharing of needles and syringes should always be avoided and as far as possible disposable one should be used.

Myth: Living with a HIV positive person could be risky as one cannot always cover one's hand and other exposed body parts.

Fact: HIV cannot be spread be touching, eating together, sharing clothes, hugging, looking after and caring for HIV positive people.

Myth: It is possible to get HIV from toilet seat.

Fact: HIV cannot be spread from toilet seats. HIV spread only through unprotected sex, infected needles, and transfusion of infected blood or from infected mother to child.

MYTH: Sharing of shaving blades in saloons can cause HIV infection.

FACT: During a shave there are chances of micro injuries and small quantity of blood may stick on the blade/razor. However, HIV is a very fragile virus, it cannot survive once exposed to sunlight. It is advisable to use a separate blade for each shave to avoid the risk of Hepatitis B and other contagious skin infections.

Myth: HIV can be transmitted by sharing cigarettes with a HIV positive person.

Fact: Saliva cannot transmit HIV; hence sharing a cigarette with a HIV positive person cannot transmit the virus.

Myth: Saliva can spread HIV infection.

Fact: Only 4 body fluids: blood, semen, vaginal fluid and breast milk are known to spread HIV if they are infected. Saliva cannot spread HIV.

Myth: Sharing food can cause HIV infection.

Fact: The mode of transmission of HIV is not the same as other infections like diarrhea; therefore, Hive infection cannot be transmitted by sharing food.

Myth: A mosquito bite can cause HIV infection if the mosquito has bitten an HIV positive person.

Fact: Mosquitoes only suck blood and do not inject blood; mosquitoes cannot spread HIV.

Myth: The result of HIV test should not be kept confidential so that other people can help the infected ones.

Fact: The shame, stigma and discrimination associated with HIV and AIDS make it important to keep the HIV test confidential.

Myth: There should be mandatory testing of HIV of all sex workers so that the spread of HIV infection can be controlled.

Fact: HIV is not spread only by sex workers. HIV testing can be done only after receiving informed consent of the person to be tested.

Myth: Any blood test can detect HIV.

Fact: No; only specific blood tests can detect the presence of HIV antibody.

Myth: The best way to known one's HIV status is by donating blood.

Fact: Donating blood is not an appropriate way to learn about one's HIV status. A HIV test should always be pre-test counseling; therefore one should go to a Voluntary Counseling & Testing Centre to get oneself tested for HIV and not to a blood bank.

Myth: HIV testing is costly affair, only few private hospitals have this facility.

Fact: HIV testing is available in almost all the Medical Government Hospitals and Voluntary Counseling & Testing Centre in India; it is free of cost.

Myth: HIV can be cured, but not AIDS.

Fact: HIV can be treated with antiretroviral drugs but cannot be cured.

Myth: Contraceptive pills can protect from inducing HIV.

Fact: No contraceptive pills can protect against HIV, as they are meant only to prevent unwanted pregnancies and not HIV.

Myth: Sex with virgin girls can protect/cure a person from HIV.

Fact: Sex with virgin girls cannot cure or protect a man from HIV.

Myth: Sex with a healthy married woman is safe.

Fact: Unprotected sex with a HIV infected person carries the risk of HIV infection, even a married woman could be infected with HIV in spite of looking healthy.

Myth: Homosexual men/gays are more prone to HIV infection.

Fact: By just being gay/homosexual will not cause HIV infection; until unprotected sex with an infected partner is there the chance of getting HIV.

Myth: Man to man sex is safe; no risk of HIV as there is any vaginal penetration.

Fact: Unprotected anal sex between men carries higher risk of HIV infection than vaginal sex; as the tissues of anal region are tighter and there are more chances of tears and cuts when penetrated and thus HIV can get very easy entry points.

Myth: If I had HIV, I'd feel sick.

Fact: Not necessarily. People can have HIV without symptoms for years. Even if a person with HIV feels good, the virus is still reproducing in the body. You may be surprised to learn that an estimated 1.2 million people are living with HIV in the United States. Of those individuals, approximately 1 in 8 do not know they are infected.

Myth: HIV only affects certain groups of people.

Fact: Anyone can get HIV—and you can become infected the first time you are exposed to the virus. HIV is spread through body fluids such as blood, semen, vaginal fluids, and breast milk. HIV is most commonly passed from one person to another through anal or vaginal sex, and by sharing needles or drug works. In addition, a mother can pass HIV to her baby during pregnancy, during labor, or through breastfeeding.

Myth: A diagnosis of HIV is a death sentence.

Fact: Although HIV is serious and there is no cure, people with HIV can now live longer, healthier lives thanks to early detection, and new and more effective treatments.

Myth: My viral load is undetectable, so I can't spread HIV.

Fact: Yes, it is possible that you could still transmit HIV. However, having an undetectable viral load greatly lowers the chance of transmitting the virus to your sexual partners who are HIV-negative. An HIV-positive person can still potentially infect a partner even if they have an undetectable viral load, because of the reasons listed below.

HIV may still be found in genital fluids (e.g., semen, vaginal fluids). The viral load test only measures virus in blood. Although antiretroviral therapy (ART) also lowers viral load in genital fluids, HIV can sometimes be present in genital fluids even when it is undetectable in the blood.

Your viral load may go up between tests. When this happens, you may be more likely to transmit HIV to sexual partners. Your viral load may go up without you knowing it because you may not feel any different.

Sexually transmitted diseases (STDs) increase viral load in genital fluids. This means that an HIV-positive person with an STD may be able to transmit HIV to sexual partners even if the blood viral load is undetectable

Myth: If I already have HIV and my partner does too, we can have unprotected sex.

Fact: You could catch another STD, such as gonorrhea, or syphilis, or another viral infection such as hepatitis C (a serious liver infection), if you don't use a condom. What you may not know is that getting another STD can increase your HIV viral load, which may speed the progression of your HIV infection. Your viral load can rise even if you're on medication for HIV (antiretroviral drugs).

Myth: My viral load is low, so I can stop taking my HIV medicines.

Fact: It is very important for you to take your HIV medicines exactly as directed. If you don't, your CD4 count may go down and your viral load many go up. When the viral load is high, risk for HIV transmission is the greatest. Even when the serum viral load is undetectable, HIV can still exist in semen, vaginal and rectal fluids, and breast milk. Taking your HIV medicine is important to help you live a longer and healthier life. Not taking your medicines as directed can also make the HIV virus resistant, which means the medicines won't help you anymore.

Myth: Because I have HIV, I should be careful about everyday activities such as sharing the telephone and shaking people's hands.

Fact: HIV cannot be caught from everyday activities, casual contact such as shaking hands, or from ordinary objects such as a doorknob, telephone, or toilet seat. The virus does not live long outside the body.

Myth: Antiretroviral drugs will cure my HIV.

Fact: Antiretroviral drugs help control reproduction of the virus and slow the progression of the disease. But they are not a cure for HIV.

Remember: It's important to take your HIV medicines exactly as your doctor tells you. If you don't, your viral load may go up. In addition, the virus may become resistant, and your medicines could stop working.

Myth: HIV treatment is too expensive.

Fact: Treatment programs and support services are available even for those who have no insurance. Medicaid is the nation's largest source of public funding for AIDS care, and the Ryan White Program provides care and support for those with limited or no health insurance.

Myth: There is a cure for HIV.

Fact: Rich or poor, there is no cure for HIV. There are ways to prolong a person's life, but once you get HIV, you will have it for the rest of your life.

Myth: If I already have HIV, I can share needles with other people who have HIV.

Fact: You shouldn't share needles, works, cottons, or water because you could get hepatitis C, a serious liver infection. Hepatitis C is one of the leading causes of chronic liver disease in the United States and hepatitis C infection progresses more rapidly to liver damage in HIV-infected persons. Outbreaks of hepatitis C have occurred among HIV-positive gay men.

Hepatitis C can result in other health problems, such as liver cancer or liver disease, which has become a major cause of hospital admissions, liver transplants, and deaths among people living with HIV. Hepatitis C infection may also impact the course and management of HIV infection. So don't share your needles, works, cottons, or water.

Myth: I only snort drugs (not shoot up), so I can share equipment without worrying about HIV.

Fact: Infected blood from inside one person's nose can be passed to another person through shared straws or other drug-snorting equipment.

So don't do it.

Myth: Getting another STD when I have HIV is no big deal.

Fact: Actually, it can be a big deal. If you have HIV, getting another infection, such as syphilis or hepatitis C, can increase your HIV viral load, which may speed the progression of your HIV infection. Your viral load can go up even if you're taking medicines for your HIV (antiretroviral drugs).

Myth: AIDS is a punishment from God. [4]

Fact: AIDS is a syndrome caused by a virus. HIV is a virus, as are the common cold and the flu. The Centers for Disease Control and Prevention and all other public health organizations stress that the AIDS epidemic is biological in nature and should be viewed as a public health concern, not a reason for judgment

Myth: Condoms are not effective at preventing HIV transmission.

Fact: When used correctly, latex and polyurethane condoms are highly effective in preventing the transmission of HIV, according to the Foundation for AIDS Research. (amfar.org). The lack of comprehensive AIDS education leads to incorrect condom usage, which greatly reduces their efficacy. Sheepskin condoms are not effective at preventing HIV transmission, as particles the size of HIV can penetrate this barrier.

Myth: Teaching comprehensive AIDS education promotes promiscuity.

Fact: Evidence shows that comprehensive sex education programs that provide information about both abstinence and contraception can help delay the onset of sexual activity among teenagers, reduce their number of sexual partners, and increase contraceptive use when they become sexually active. These findings were underscored in "Call to Action to Promote Sexual Health and Responsible Sexual Behavior," issued by former Surgeon General David Satcher in June 2001.

Myth: AIDS started from sexual intercourse with monkeys.

Fact: HIV is a mutated form of SIV, simian immunodeficiency virus According to the Centers for Disease Control and Prevention, scientists best explanation is that the virus was able to cross species due to repeated contact of hunters with infected blood from chimpanzees. The origin of HIV is far less important than our response to the current global epidemic.

Myth: Packaged condoms, medications, and other inanimate objects can contain HIV.

Fact: HIV can only live in human blood, semen, vaginal fluid, and breast milk, and dies once these fluids have dried. HIV can only be transmitted via direct contact with one of these fluids. According to the Centers for Disease Control and Prevention, HIV cannot live outside of the body (except in carefully controlled laboratory settings) making HIV transmission from packaged condoms or other items impossible.

Chapter 6

MEDICAL ASSESSMENT OF HIV INFECTED PATIENT

Dr. Sunita Pathak

Successful treatment of HIV infected patients depends on proper medical assessment. The main concerns for the dental practitioner are bleeding, infections and drug interactions. An appropriate medical assessment will help prevent complications from dental therapy as well as aid the diagnosis of oral lesions.

TRANSMISSION CATEGORY

This transmission category includes homosexual or bisexual men, injection drug users, hemophiliacs, recipients of blood products and those who acquired HIV through heterosexual contact.

DATE OF INITIAL INFECTION & HIV TEST

The date of initial infection is very hard to ascertain in most patients except for infections that are acquired congenitally or through blood transfusions. The time of infection is the best predictor for disease progression. To approximate the time of initial infection, it is advantageous to obtain the date of patient's 1st positive HIV test result and the reason the patient was tested.

HISTORY OF SEXUALLY TRANSMITTED DISEASE

Patients with HIV and a history of multiple sexually transmitted diseases show a faster progression of HIV disease. Herpes simplex virus infection, gonorrhea and syphilis are the most common STD's reported among this group of patients.

HISTORY OF INFECTIOUS DISEASE

Concurrent infections with HBV and HIV may occur in over 90% of HIV infected individuals. However liver damage in patients with concurrent chronic HBV infection and AIDS appears to be less severe than that in patients without HIV infection, despite the fact that a higher incidence of HBeAg expression is noted among homosexual men with HIV compared to homosexual men without HIV. Consequently, HBV infection in homosexual men with HIV may indicate a more contagious state but cause less liver damage. Hepatic manifestations in HIV disease are usually associated with drug toxicity, hepatitis C virus or hepatitis D virus infection. The incidence of HCV infection in HIV infected patients is estimated to be approximately 7%. Tuberculosis is the only major opportunistic infection that may be contagious to immune competent health-care workers. Dental providers need to recognize the typical signs and symptoms associated with TB like productive cough, cough with blood in the sputum, chest pain, fever, night sweats, weight loss and malaise.

PAST AND PRESENT HIV RELATED OPPTURNISTIC INFECTION

Past and present HIV related opportunistic infections may indicate what type of medications the patient is taking as well as HIV status and staging. A patient's HIV associated medications usually indicate past and/ or present infections and suggest possible hematologic abnormalities and sometimes immune status. Antiretroviral drugs are solely used in patients with HIV. These patients must be assessed for increased bleeding tendencies, by evaluating platelet counts and for increased susceptibility to infections by evaluating neutrophil counts. Patients with histories of drug allergies tend to have a high incidence of allergic reactions toward more than one medication. The administrations of medications ordinarily used for oral infections in patients without HIV is usually not contraindicated for patients with HIV. Patients with reduced gastric secretions should not be given medications that are activated by gastric acid such as ketoconazole or dapsone. Furthermore, patients with severe diarrhea and wasting syndrome will not be able to efficiently absorb oral medications. Overall medications should be administered only if there is a clear medical indication. An increased number of medications may cause unanticipated adverse drug interactions.

ALLERGIES

During the progression of HIV disease patients show an increased susceptibility to developing drug allergies. This is a curious occurrence since drug reactions are usually associated with an intact T-lymphocyte response. Therefore, reduced allergic reaction would be expected in individuals with advanced HIV disease.

TOBACCO AND ALCOHOL USE

Tobacco smoking has not been associated with immune impairment in individuals with HIV. Instead, an increased white blood cell count has been documented in smokers during the earliest stages of HIV disease. However heavy smokers may be at higher risk for developing opportunistic pneumonias. The consumption of alcohol drinking increases and may augment HIV replication. Chronic alcoholism has also been associated with profound depression of T-suppressor lymphocyte function. Patients who continue to use injection drugs need to be counseled. This habit will enhance HIV disease progression in the drug user and may put other persons at risk.

SOCIAL SUPPORT SYSTEM

Many oral manifestations are early signs of HIV disease and AIDS. Therefore, a dentist may have to inform a patient that he or she has clinical indications of HIV disease. It is essential that the dental providers refer the patient to appropriate support networks in the patient's geographic area. It is also pertinent to inquire about a patient's personal support system. These people usually offer the most valuable support to the patient, but only if the patient is accepted by them.

LABORATORY VALUES

Laboratory values indicate hemostasis and risk of infection, two of the most common concerns affecting the provision of dental care. However, with HIV infected patients the dental providers also need to pay special attention to the patient's overall immune status. Patients with absolute neutrophil counts below 500 cells/mm^3 should receive antibiotic prophylaxis prior to dental therapy. A progressive decrease in CD4+ cell counts is the hallmark of HIV disease. Indications of a patient's prognosis are usually based on absolute CD4+ cell counts or CD4%.

REVIEW OF SYSTEMIC SYSTEMS

The dissemination of HIV within different body systems, as well as the associated immune deterioration create specific manifestations throughout the body.

1) Head & Neck

Sinusitis appears to be a common complication of HIV disease. The incidence and severity of sinusitis increased with progression of HIV disease. The high incidence of dry mouth in patients with HIV may be partially explained by mouth breathing and xerostomia inducing medications associated with chronic sinusitis. Past and present episodes of epistaxis indicate possible bleeding abnormalities. Persistent generalized lymphadenopathy occurs commonly in the cervical lymph nodes of individuals with HIV and is characterized by lymph nodes approximately 10mm in diameter, rubbery to hard and usually freely movable.

2) Gastrointestinal tract

Diarrhoea and malabsorption both play an important part in the development of wasting syndrome in HIV infected individuals. A progressive loss of lean body mass can be seen in patients with AIDS. Nutritional deficiencies will also impair the immune response. Reduction of T lymphocytes, impaired cell mediated immune response, reduced natural killer cell activity and altered phagocytic functions have all been associated with nutritional deficiencies. Vitamin B_{12} malabsorption is not uncommon in patients with HIV and may initially present as an oral manifestation. Patients with HIV may have undergone splenectomies as treatment for immune thrombocytopenia purpura should also be evaluated.

3) Cardiac system

The true incidence of cardiac involvement in HIV disease is not clear. Cardiomyopathy can be caused by a wide variety of opportunistic infections associated with HIV infection.

4) Pulmonary system

Pneumocytis carinii pneumonia is by far most common type of pulmonary disease in patients with AIDS. P. carinii pneumonitis isan AIDS diagnosis in HIV infected individuals and is usually only found in patients with severe immune suppression. Identification of patients with TB becomes essential to treat the patient with appropriate precautions and facilitate referrals for medical treatment.

5) Neurologic manifestations

Patients with AIDS may exhibit signs of HIV encephalopathy which is associated with decreased motor and cognitive abilities. This type of patients may have difficulties performing normal oral hygiene procedures, forget appointments and have an unstable mental status.

Chapter 7

INFECTION CONTROL

Dr. Vishal Mehrotra
Dr. Vinayak Rai

Infection control involves the prevention of the passage of infectious disease from the patient to health care providers and other patients who may be subsequently treated in the same area. It also involves the prevention of transmission of any additional infectious disease to the already compromised patient, such as HIV infected patients.

Preventing the transmission of infectious disease from patients to health care worker has always been a concern. It became of major importance with the rising numbers of in the general population who became infected with hepatitis B virus, genital herpes viruses and HIV. The infection control program for the special patients is strict adherence to these currently promulgated standards and guidelines, called universal precautions. They are called universal because they are to be applied to all patients and all treatment procedures. These infection control guidelines include appropriate procedures to protect all dental patients as well as all dental care providers from the hazard of infectious disease transmission in the dental office.

IMMUNIZATION AGAINST HEPATITIS B VIRUS

All personnel in the dental office, including the receptionist should be antibody positive for the hepatitis B virus. The employer must provide the vaccine at no cost to the employee as required by Occupational Health and Safety Administration. Each vaccine recipient should be tested 2 or 3 months after the series of injections is complete.

BARRIER TECHNIQUES

The proper use of barrier techniques as part of universal precautions is extremely important. The wearing of gloves, masks, protective eyewear and clinic attire by all personnel who have direct patient contact is required for all treatment sessions, regardless of their nature.

1) Gloving and Handwashing

Hands must be washed carefully with an antiseptic lotion soap that has persistent antibacterial activities. Hands should be dried thoroughly and a lotion applied to help maintain healthy skin. Gloves are changed for each patient, when they are damaged or torn or if the procedure extends longer than 1hour. To avoid cross-contamination special care should be taken to avoid touching items with the gloved hands that are not directly in the field of operation, including the patient care record, progress slips, pencils, computer keyboards, radiographs and amalgamators.

2) Mask

Masks should have at least 95% filtration efficiency for particles 3.0 to 5.0 micrometer in diameter and they should be changed for each patient. A chin length face shield may be worn in addition to the mask for greater protection against particular splatter.

3) Protective eyewear

Protective eyewear with side eyeshields should be worn by dental team all the time of dental procedure of HIV infected patients.

4) Clinic Attire

Appropriate clinic attire provides protective covering for street clothing and exposed skin. This is especially important for individuals who participate directly in patient treatment to avoid contamination by infectious aerosols and splatter. Gowns that have been worn during treatment of patients should be removed before leaving the office or while eating. The clinic cloth should be laundered in hot water, with bleach in the fabric.

5) Hair Control

All personnel involved in direct patient care should take steps to assure that hair does not come into contact with equipment or supplies used in patient care or intrude into the treatment field. Disposable caps are available at dental or medical supply houses and may be worn for routine patient care if desired.

STERILIZATION

Each dental office must properly clean, disinfect and sterilize all instruments and equipment used in the treatment of one patient before it is used with another patients.

1) Cleaning of instruments

The removal of gross organic soil (bioburden) ie:saliva, blood and residues of dental restorative material, before attempting a sterilization process is extremely important. The simplest and safest method for accomplishing this cleaning process is with an ultrasonic cleaner. Instruments are rinsed free of gross debris in the operatory, but scrubbing with a brush is neither necessary nor desirable since this could result in injury to the health care worker. A presoak solution prevents the bioburden from drying on the instruments and allows the cleaning process to remove it easily.

2) Heat sterilization

Various methods are followed like steam autoclave;is the instrument of choice for sterilization if there are many cloth or paper wrapped packs to deal with such as those found in the offices of periodontists and oral surgeons. Chemiclave is another method works well with single- or double-layer wraps such as the mylar and paper tubing or pouches. Process indicators take the form of colored printing on the wrap or a striped piece of tape on the package. If a color change takes place, it indicates that the package was processed in the sterilizer.

DISINFECTION

It is a chemical process whereby the total numbers of microbes are reduced in number, but may not be totally eliminated. The surfaces to be cleaned and disinfected should be sprayed until they glisten and then thoroughly wiped with a paper towel moistened with the disinfectant to remove the gross contamination. The solution should be sprayed a second time and allowed to remain on the surface for the recommended time. Chemicals that are acceptable for disinfection of environmental surfaces include aqueous iodophor solutions, combined synthetic phenolics, phenol-alcohol sprays and sodium hypochloride solution diluted 1:5 to 1:100.

OPERATORY MANAGEMENT

1) The removal of extraneous items

The removal of extraneous items from treatment rooms is important because of the fallout of bacterial aerosols and gross splash and splatter that constantly occur. Removing the bulk storage containers and substituting 'unit dose' amounts of each item in small packets is simple. In place of cotton roll dispenser 4or5 cotton rolls may be placed in a small envelope, stapled if a steam autoclave will be used to sterilize them or simply sealed if a chemiclave is the preferred method of sterilization. Restorative material should be brought from the central supply area as needed, in procedure tubes with all the necessary materials and supplies for a specific dental treatment and handled with freshly washed hands or gloves. The burs required for each treatment are packaged and sterilized in the instrument's setup on a small bur block or the new single use disposable burs are used.

2) Between Patient Appointments

These activities are divided into removal, cleaning and disinfection and resetting:

a) Removal –

- Remove the drape from the patient and use it to cover the instruments on the setup tray.
- Done utility gloves

- Remove the handpieces from the unit and put them on the tray with the contaminated instruments for removal to the central sterilization area, so that they must be properly cleaned and wrapped for sterilization.
- Remove the headrest cover, disposable saliva ejector, high velocity evacuator and three-way syringe tips and place them in the trash bag on the cabinet.
- Place in the trash bag attached to the mobile cabinet any other patient-contaminated waste remaining on the cabinet top as well as the used patient towel which has been used to cover the instrument during dismissal.
- Remove the trash bag from the cabinet, twist it tightly to enclose the debris, cycle it through the heat sterilizer if required in one's area and dispose of it in the properly marked waste receptacle.

b) Cleaning and disinfection-

- Wash the utility gloved hands properly disinfect any items remaining on the cabinet top with the spray, wipe and spray technique and return them to their proper place in the cabinet drawers.
- Heat sterilizes the handpiece and is packaged and processed through the sterilizer. A lubricant is sprayed into the drive airline before the handpiece is connected to the air line.
- If the unit reaches to the sink, run a large volume of water through each evacuation and saliva ejector hose by passing the handles back and forth through a stream of running water.
- Spray with disinfectant and wipe the cabinet top, drawer handles, light handles, chair switch buttons, top of unit, three-way syringe and evacuator handles and handpiece hoses.
- Rinse dental impressions immediately on removal from the mouth to remove all blood and saliva. Then immerse them in an acceptable disinfectant solution and take them to the laboratory for casting.

c) Seating the patient and resetting the operatory-

- Seat the patient, dental workers should adjust their mask and protective eyewear, wash their hands with the antibacterial lotion soap and put on fresh gloves. Place a disposable saliva ejector tip and high velocity evacuator tip. Open the sealed pouch containing the sterilized handpiece, partially remove it and lubricate it. Set up on the controller and run water through handpiece for 30sec before connecting the handpiece.
- Ask the patient to rinse their mouth with an antibacterial mouthwash prior to the procedure.
- Attach the trash bag to a convenient location on the edge of back or side or edge of cart.
- From the procedure tub or tubs brought from the central sterilization area assemble the required armamentaria on the covered tray.

COVERS AND DISPOSABLES

It is easier to prevent contamination with the proper use of covers than it is to decontaminate a soiled surface. And it is more certain to prevent contamination than to assume that the disinfection process will totally kill any organisms that have accumulated on the uncovered surface. Uses of covers could include the newly introduced finger cots for slow speed handpieces and ultrasonic scaler handles. Products that are purchased for single use are not intended to be sterilized and reused. It is not safe to try to clean and disinfect these items for reuse. Properly cleaning, lubricating and sterilizing by heat a prophy angle after each use can consume a considerable amount of time.

CENTRAL STERILIZATION AREA

It is recommended that the processes of cleaning and sterilizing dental instruments be carried out in an area devoted to that sole purpose. The movement of instruments should be in a flow pattern that does not require clean materials and contaminated items to cross paths.

a) Cleaning of instruments

Thorough cleaning of recyclable instruments must precede any efforts at sterilization. Bioburden must be removed. A twostep process is followed: a container should be on or near the field of operation in the treatment room and it should contain either a disinfectant or a detergent solution. When an instrument has been used for the last time in the procedure, simply place it in the liquid in the container. When the patient is dismissed the container along with all the other contaminated articles may be removed from the treatment room to the central sterilization area for handling. When it is time to clean the instrument, the liquid should be poured into the sink and the instruments placed into the ultrasonic cleaner.[74]

WASTE CONTROL

To comply with CDC, ADA & OSHA guidelines needles and other sharps must be disposed of in a hard walled puncture proof container as close to the point of use as possible. We should not bend or break needles but dispose of them in sharps container that allow the removal of the needle without the hazard of recapping by hand. If recapping must be done, the cap must be placed in a holder or held in a hemostat or use the one handed swoop technique to put the point of the needle in the cap then rinse the syringe to a vertical position and allow the cap to settle down over the needle. Cotton rolls 2x2 gauze, patient towels and other items that have absorbed patient secretions during treatment may be considered contaminated or infectious waste, depending on the area in which one's practice is located. If this patient contaminated waste must be handled differently from common trash it can be handled easily if a small bag is attached to the cabinet or unit for each patient. Place all the patient contaminated waste into this bag as it is generated and heat sterilize it.[74]

BIBLIOGRAPHY

1. Alison L. Drake et al. Herpes Simplex Virus Type 2 and Risk of Intrapartum Human Immunodeficiency Virus Transmission. Obstetrics & Gynecology Feb 2007,109,2 (1):403-9.
2. Amit Chattopadhyay et al. Incidence of Oral Candidiasis and Oral Hairy Leukoplakia in HIV-infected adults in North Carolina. Oral Surg Oral Med Oral Pathol Oral Radiol Endod 2005;99:25-47.
3. Adler-Storthz K,Ficarra G,Woods KV,Gaglioti D,DiPietro M,Shillitoe EJ. Prevalence of Epstein Barr virus and human papillomavirus in oral mucosa of HIV infected patients. Journal of Oral Pathol Med 1992;21:164-70
4. Burket's Oral Medicine,Diagnosis and Treatment. 10ed 2003:538-56.
5. Connie L Celum,Noah J.Robinson and Myron S.Cohen. Potential Effect of HIV type-1 antiretroviral and herpes simplex virus type-2 antiviral therapy on transmission and acquisition of HIV type-1 infection. The Journal of Infectious Disease 2005;191(suppl-1):S107-14
6. Centers for disease control and prevention. Human immunodeficiency virus type-2. 1998: 1-4.
7. HIV/AIDS Myths and Facts
8. 8 Common Myths About HIV and Aids
9. **cdc.gov/Features/LetsStopHIV**
10. **cdc.gov/actagainstaids/campaigns/ starttalking**
11. 13 Facts and Myths about HIV and AIDS - Children for Health
12. AIDS Misinformation in 2025: Myths, Facts, and How to Respond - AIDS.org
13. hiv-myths-and-facts-booklet.pdf
14. Centers for disease control and prevention.Human immunodeficiency virus type-2.1998: 1-4.

15. Chaudhry Z,Barrett AW,Corbett E,French PD,Zakrzewska JM. Oral mucosal leishmaniasis as a presenting feature of HIV infection and its management. Journal of Oral Pathol Med 1999;28:43-6.

16. Centers for disease control and prevention.HIV and its transmission.1999:1-4.

17. Harals E.Fischer.Human Immunodeficiency virus type-2:implications for Blood Donors.Current issues in transfusion medicine 1993

18. Hoosen M Coovadia et al. Mother to child transmission of HIV-1 infection during exclusive breastfeeding in the first 6months of life: an intervention cohort study. Lancet 2007;369:1107-1115.

19. Ivan D.Miziara. Tuberculosis affecting the oral cavity in Brazillian HIV infected patients. Oral Surg Oral Med Oral Pathol Oral Radiol Endod 2005;100:179-82.

20. Jair C.Leao et al. Cheilitis glandularis: An unusual presentation in a patient with HIV infection. Oral Surg Oral Med Oral Pathol Oral Radiol Endod 2003;95:142-4.

21. Louis Mandel and Farisa Surattanont. Regression of HIV parotid swellings after retroviral therapy: Case reports with computed tomographic scan evidence. Oral Surg Oral Med Oral Pathol Oral Radiol Endod 2002;94:454-9.

22. LL.Patton et al.Prevalence and classification of HIV associated oral lesions. Oral Disease 2002;8(2):98-109.

23. Mark W.Kline. Perspectives on the Pediatric HIV/AIDS pandemic: Catalyzing Acssess of Children to care and treatment. Pediatrics 2006;117:1388-1393.

24. Melissa Miller et al. Breast milk erythropoietin and mother-to-child HIV transmission through breastmilk. Lancet 2002;360(19):1246-48.

25. Scully C et al. Detection of Epstein-bar virus in oral scrapes in HIV infection, in hairy leukoplakia, and in healthy non-HIV-infected people.

J Oral Pathol Med 1998;27:480-2.

26. Syrjanen S et al. Oral hairy leukoplakia is not a specific sign of HIV-infection but related to immunosuppression in general.J Oral Pathol Med 1989; 18: 28-31

27. Sporri B et al. Reduced nuber of langerhans cells in oral mucosal washings from HIV-1 seropositives. J Oral Pathol Med 1994; 23: 399-402.

28. Warnakulasuriya KAAS et al. Localized oral histoplasmosis lesions associated with HIV infection. J Oral Pathol Med 1997;26:294-6

29. Wanzala P et al. Low prevalence of oral mucosal lesions in HIV-1 seropositive African women. J Oral Pathol Med 1989;18:416-418

30. Zhang X et al. Ultrastructural findings in oral hyperpigmentation of HIV-infected patients. J Oral Pathol Med 1989;18:471-426

31. Zhang X et al Ultrastructural findings in clinically uninvolved oral mucosa of patients with HIV infection. J Oral Pathol Med 1989;18:35-4